# The Complete KETO Snack Cookbook For Women

Healthy And Delicious Keto-Friendly Snacks For Weight Loss

*Megan Kelly*

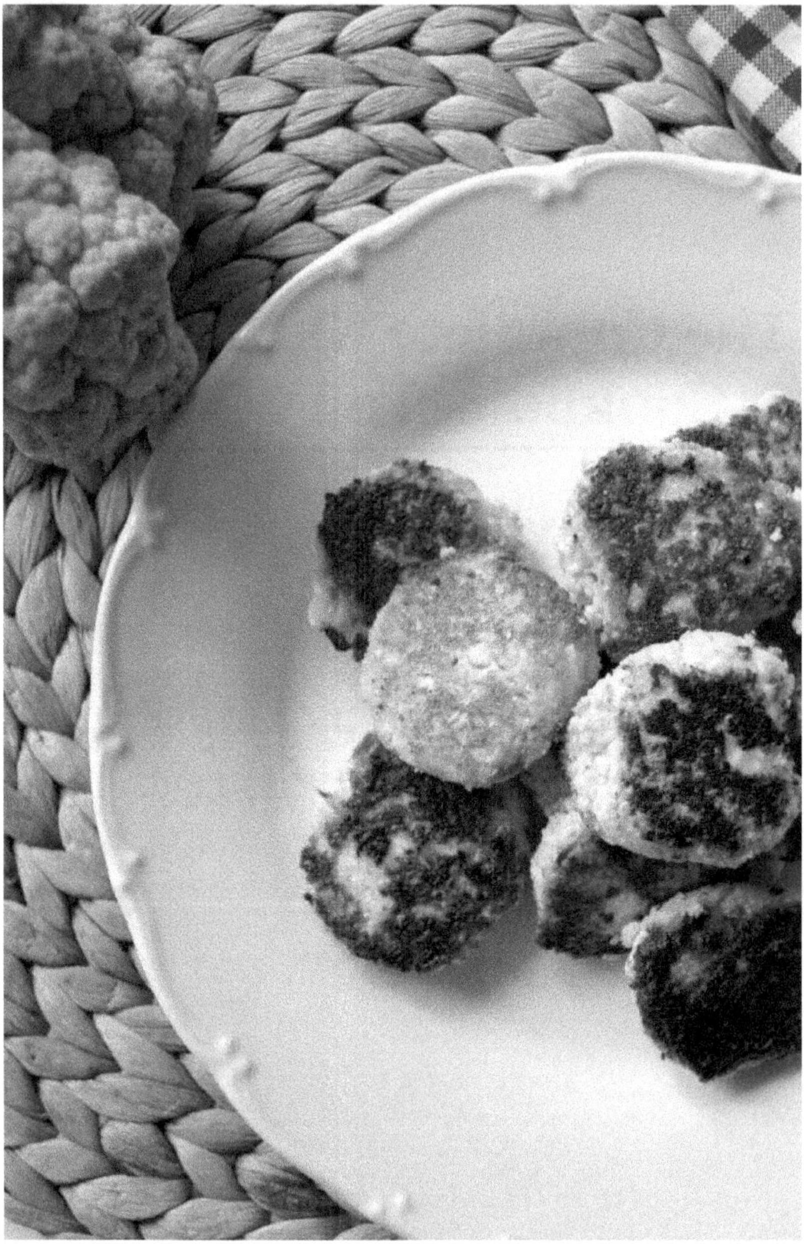

# Table of contents

# Braised Escarole with Onions

**Servings:** 4

**Time:** 25 mins

**Difficulty:** Easy

**Nutrients per serving:** Calories: 124 kcal | Fat: 11g | Carbohydrates: 7g | Protein: 2g | Fiber: 4g

## Ingredients

- vinegar of your choice
- Freshly ground black pepper
- Diamond Crystal kosher salt
- 3 tbsp olive oil or ghee
- 1 onion thinly sliced
- 1 large head of escarole ~2 lb
- 1 garlic clove minced

## Method

1. The first thing you have to do is isolate and wash the escarole leaves properly (lots of mud and dust can be

there at the base of these inner leaves). Drain and cut coarsely.

2. Heat the ghee over medium heat in a large skillet and sauté the onions until tender. Throw the garlic in and stir for about 30 seconds and then pour the escarole in it (damp greens are acceptable).
3. The greens and the onions are finely salted and cooked until the leaves are wilted and soft (about 12-15 minutes). Add salt and pepper to season, and add a dash of your preferred vinegar.

# Keto Cheese Chips

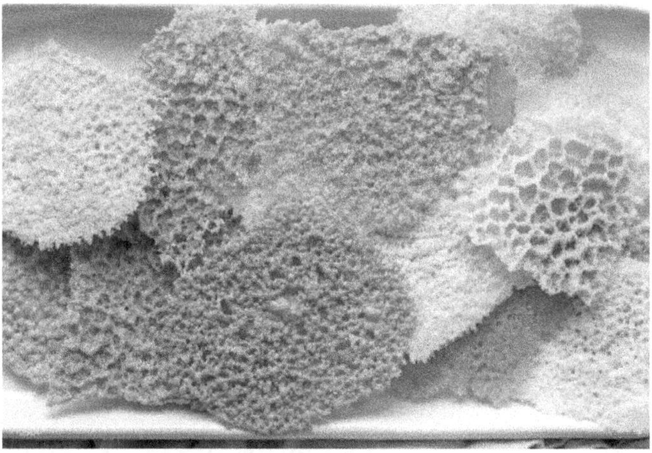

**Servings:** 6

**Time:** 18 mins

**Difficulty:** Easy

**Nutrients per serving:** Calories: 74 kcal | Fat: 4.88g| Carbohydrates: 0.61g | Protein: 6.76g

## Ingredients

- Herbs, spices, spice blends
- 4 oz Parmesan Cheese

## Method

1. Preheat the oven to 400 °F. Put the rack in the center position. Line the parchment paper with a large baking sheet. If you don't have a grated Parmesan, process the cheese into fine crumbles.
2. Measure the tspful of cheese and put it on a parchment-lined Panipat every mound of cheese softly (about 1 1/4 to 1 1/2 inches) in a circle with a finger. Until baking, dust with any herbs, sauces, or flavorings.
3. Cook the Parmesan crisps for 6 to 8 minutes before they begin to turn golden brown. Let it cool fully for up to 30 days before storing; put it in an airtight jar for about a week or in the fridge.

# Rosemary Roasted Rutabaga

**Servings:** 4

**Time:** 45 mins

**Difficulty:** Easy

**Nutrients per serving:** Calories: 100 kcal | Fat: 6.51g | Carbohydrates: 10g | Protein: 1.47g | Fiber: 3g

## Ingredients

- 1 lb Rutabaga (peeled and cut into the 3/4-inch cubes)
- 1/8 tsp Freshly ground pepper
- 1/4 cup diced onion (1 oz)
- 1/4 tsp Salt
- 1 tbsp Chopped fresh rosemary
- 1 tbsp Olive oil
- 1 tbsp butter or ghee

## Method

1. Preheat the oven to 400 °F. Put the rack in the center. Using parchment paper to cover a sheet pan.

2. Toss the onion, olive oil, pepper, rosemary, salt with the cubed rutabaga and spread it uniformly over the sheet pan. Bake about 20-30 minutes or until tender with a fork.
3. Over lower heat, heat a medium to the large frying pan. Apply the butter and swirl when heated to coat the plate. Fry a rutabaga until browned lightly.
4. To eliminate additional carbs, serve with fried, pan-seared, or roasted meat and a side salad.

# Oven-Fried Parmesan Green Beans

**Servings:** 6

**Time:** 30 mins

**Difficulty:** Easy

**Nutrients per serving:** Calories: 133 kcal | Fat: 9.88g | Carbohydrates: 6.19g | Protein: 5.3g | Fiber: 2.7g

## Ingredients

Parmesan Green Beans

- 1/4 tsp salt
- 1/2 cup Parmesan cheese (Kraft in the can is fine)
- 1 lb green beans (stem end trimmed and dried with paper towels)
- 1 tsp minced garlic
- 1 large egg white (whipped until very frothy)

Sweet Mustard Dipping Sauce

- 1/4 cup mayonnaise (4 tbsp)
- 1/4 tsp dried dill, rubbed (or tarragon)
- 1/4 tsp pepper
- 1 1/2 tsp yellow mustard
- 1/2 tsp garlic salt

- 1/2 tsp smoked paprika (or regular)
- 2 tbsp sweetener of choice

## Method

1. Preheat the oven to 425 °F. Put the rack in the center spot. Using parchment paper to cover a large baking dish.
2. In a shallow cup, mix these Parmesan cheese & minced garlic, and 1/4 tsp salt.
3. In a large cup, put the green beans and toss with the white egg until fully coated. Add the combination of cheese and toss to cover.
4. On the parchment-lined baking dish, scatter the green beans and sprinkle any leftover cheese on top.
5. Bake around 15-20 minutes or unless the beans become cooked and browned with the cheese.
6. Mix the ingredients for Sweet Mustard Sauce as the beans cook.

# Crispy Pepperoni Chips

**Servings:** 1

**Time:** 13 mins

**Difficulty:** Easy

**Nutrients per serving:** Calories: 150 kcal | Fat: 14g | Carbohydrates: 1g | Protein: 5g

## Ingredients

- 15 Pre-sliced pepperoni slices (about one inch in diameter)

## Method

Oven/Toaster Oven:

1. Preheat the oven to 400 °F. 375 F for the toaster oven and place the rack in the center. Line parchment on a sheet pan. Put the pepperoni on a parchment, spread them evenly or if you're filling the sheet pan, let them just hit.

2. Bake for 4 minutes. Be careful not to damage yourself with a paper towel—Bake for a further 4 minutes or until slightly browned with pepperoni. On a paper towel, remove and rinse.

Microwave:

1. Place the pepperoni on the paper towel on a healthy microwave plate and cook until crispy, at the interval of 20 seconds. Since microwaves differ in strength and wattage, the approximate time will rely on your microwave.

# Tangy Ranch Chicken Wings

**Servings:** 4

**Time:** 1 hr

**Difficulty:** Easy

**Nutrients per serving:** Calories: 341 kcal | Fat: 27.8g | Carbohydrates: 3g | Protein: 26g | Fiber: 2.4g

## Ingredients

- Olive oil spray
- 2 tsp olive oil
- 2 tsp Baking Powder
- 2 lb Chicken wing pieces
- 2 1/2 tsp Homemade Ranch Seasoning
- 1/4 tsp Salt

## Method

1. Preheat the oven to 375 °F with the middle rack in place.
2. Dry the chicken wings with paper towels and place them in a wide dish.

3. Mix 2 tsp of olive oil with the chicken wings once seasoned. Sprinkle the baking powder with 1 tsp and blend. Only repeat.
4. Place the chicken wings over a wide sheet pan and skin-side-up on a wire rack. Bake the chicken for 40 minutes, flipping it halfway through.
5. Take the chicken out of the oven and turn it upside-down again, for about 5-10 minutes just until the chicken is browned and crispy and put under the broiler.
6. Take a big bowl of chicken and gently brush it with olive oil. Over the chicken, sprinkle 1 tsp of ranch seasoning and stir to cover. Repeat with the seasoning, but add 1/4 of a tsp of salt. Just serve.

# Cabbage Noodles

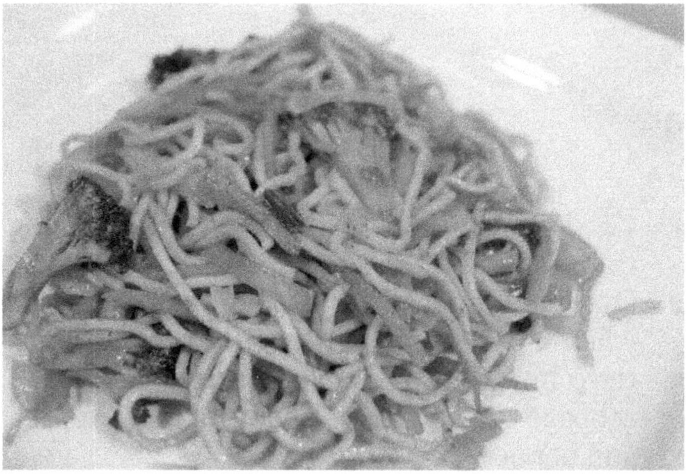

**Servings:** 4

**Time:** 20 mins

**Difficulty:** Easy

**Nutrients per serving:** Calories: 82 kcal | Fat: 5.9g | Carbohydrates: 7.3g | Protein: 1.8g | Fiber: 2.7g

## Ingredients

- 1/4 cup onions, sliced thinly (1 oz)
- 1 lb cabbage (cored and cut into strips)

- 2 cloves garlic, sliced
- 2 tbsp butter or oil
- salt and pepper to taste

## Method

1. Cut into quarters of the cabbage. Slice the onions thinly and peel the garlic.
2. Over medium fire, heat a skillet. Apply the butter or oil when it is scorching and swirl to cover the plate. Add the cabbage, garlic, and onion and then saute until the cabbage becomes soft - about 10 minutes—salt to taste and pepper.

# Oatmeal Sugar-Free Cookies

**Servings:** 20

**Time:** 29 mins

**Difficulty:** Easy

**Nutrients per serving:** Calories: 119 kcal | Fat: 11.3g | Carbohydrates: 2.94g | Protein: 3.2g | Fiber: 1.8g

## Ingredients

- 3/4 tsp cinnamon
- 1/4 tsp baking soda
- 1/4 tsp salt
- 1/3 cup Low carbohydrate brown sugar (50 g)
- 1/2 tsp of vanilla extract
- 1 1/2 cups sliced almonds (5 oz/142 g)
- 4 oz unsalted butter, softened (113 g)
- 1 cup of almond flour (95 g)
- 1 large egg, cold (room temperature)
- 2 tbsp of oat fiber (10 g)
- 2 tsp of grass-fed beef gelatin

**Method**

1. Preheat the oven to 350 °F. Put the rack in the center position. Line parchment on a sheet pan. In a food processor or just by hand, cut sliced almonds to imitate the size of oats. Quantify and stir together the dry ingredients to remove the lumps.
2. Sukrin Gold, vanilla extract, and Butter softened together until they become light and fluffy - around 1 1/2 minutes. Scrape the bowl down.
3. At once, add all the dry ingredients and beat until mixed. Include the egg, and beat until mixed. The cut sliced almonds fold in.
4. Scoop the dough and put on the baking sheet two inches apart using the 2 tbsp cookie scoop.
5. Bake for 8 minutes, take from the oven, and softly bang a cookie sheet on the oven or counter to flatten the cookies - about 6 times. Keep in the oven for an extra 6 minutes.
6. Take the cookies from the oven and use the spatula to slap each cookie gently. Before removing them from the cooling rack, let them cool for around 5 minutes. Until eating it, again cool these thoroughly.

# Pulled Pork Stuffed Avocado Boats

**Servings:** 4

**Time:** 15 mins

**Difficulty:** Easy

**Nutrients per serving:** Calories: 423 kcal | Fat: 34g | Carbohydrates: 9g | Protein: 23.5g | Fiber: 5g

## Ingredients

- 1/4 cup BBQ sauce
- 1 1/2 cups pork or chicken (pulled)
- 2 avocados, halved and pitted

Garnish

- 1 tbsp snipped chives or green onion
- 2 tbsp BBQ sauce (sugar -free)
- 2 tbsp ranch dressing (thinned slightly)

## Method

1. Halve the avocados and drain the pit. To make space for the filling, scoop out some of the avocados. (You may mash it and blend it or put it on the top of pulled pork with a ranch dressing. I gave it to the children.)
2. In a microwave or the frying pan, heat the pulled pork, and mix it with 1/4 cup of BBQ sauce of your choice. Dispense equally between the halves of the avocado.
3. Drizzle each half with the remaining ranch dressing and BBQ sauce. Add chives or green onion to garnish.
4. You can eat as it is or pop put it in the microwave to warm it. Alternatively, put in a 350 F preheated oven and bake for around 20 minutes, sealed. Cover some leftovers and refrigerate them.

# Sweet Bell Pepper Salad

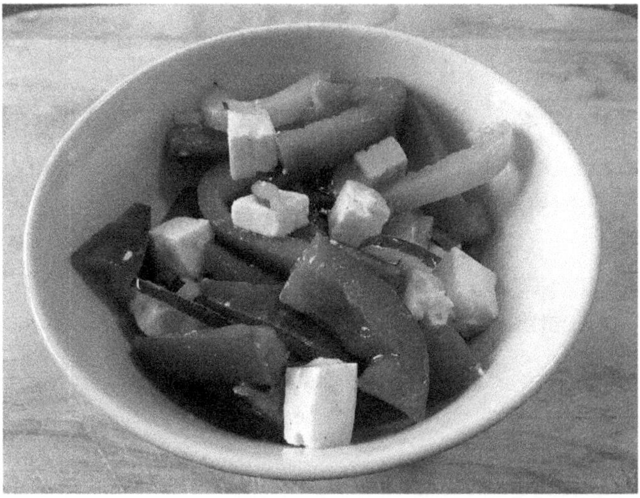

**Servings:** 6

**Time:** 15 mins

**Difficulty:** Easy

**Nutrients per serving:** Calories: 112 kcal | Fat: 9g | Carbohydrates: 6.4g | Protein: 2g | Fiber: 2g

**Ingredients**

- 2 oz feta cheese crumbled
- 2 oz. onion, sliced thinly

- 1/2 tsp garlic, minced
- 1 lb mixed bell peppers, sliced
- 1 fennel bulb, sliced thinly

Dressing

- 1 pinch pepper
- 1/2 tsp Fines Herbs (basil, tarragon, parsley, dill)
- 1/4 tsp salt
- 2 tbsp Champagne vinegar (you can also use rice wine vinegar)
- 3 tbsp extra virgin olive oil

**Method**

1. Cut and soak each onion in 1/4 cup of water and 2 tbsp of white vinegar for 10-15 minutes if you use heavy onions. Drain, use, again.
2. Cut the vegetables into a medium-large serving bowl and add them.
3. Mix up the dressing ingredients. Ensure that the fines herbs are rubbed on your palm or rubbed on your fingers to crack the flavor to extract it.
4. To change the seasoning, toss, and taste. Apply the cheese to the feta and toss gently. Only serve it cold.

# Keto Baba Ganoush

**Servings:** 8

**Time:** 55 mins

**Difficulty:** Easy

**Nutrients per serving:** Calories: 81 kcal | Fat: 6g | Carbohydrates: 6.3g | Protein: 2.3g | Fiber: 3.3g

## Ingredients

- 1/4 cup Greek yogurt
- 1 large eggplant, sliced lengthwise (1 1/2 lb)
- 2 tsp minced garlic (1-2 cloves)
- 1/2 tsp ground cumin
- 2 tbsp tahini paste
- 2 tbsp extra virgin olive oil
- 1 tbsp lemon juice
- salt and pepper to taste

## Method

1. Preheat the oven to 400°F. Please put it in the middle spot on the oven rack. Using parchment paper to cover a sheet pan.
2. Lengthwise, slice the eggplant, salt generously, and leave to rest for 15 minutes to remove the bitter juices. Quickly scrub, then pat dry. When pierced with a fork, put the eggplant having cut side down, then roast for 45 minutes or when the eggplant is fully tender. Remove and cool from the oven
3. Scoop the skin from the soft eggplant pulp and put it in a food processor. Now Pulse to split-up. Include the other ingredients and process until the dip becomes smooth and creamy in the blender.
4. Taste the seasoning and adjust. Serve right away, or cover and refrigerate for up to five days. The next day it tastes better. Serve mildly warm like room temperature.

# Low Carb Keto Taco Shells

**Servings:** 6

**Time:** 25 mins

**Difficulty:** Easy

**Nutrients per serving:** Calories: 171 kcal | Fat: 13.6g | Carbohydrates: 1g | Protein: 10.6g

## Ingredients

- 9 oz pre-shredded cheddar cheese

## Method

1. Put one rack in the upper third and the other rack in the lower third of the oven and preheat the oven to 375 $^{o}$F. Using parchment paper to cover two wide sheet pans. (Flip the parchment over so that the cheese doesn't have a pencil or pen.)
2. Quantify 1/3 cup (1 1/2 ounce) per circle of shredded cheese and spread uniformly over the sides of the circle.

3. Bake about 5 minutes and swap the baking sheets' places. Bake for another 5-10 minutes, or until the cheese layer has small holes and the edges tend to tan.
4. Before removing onto wooden spoons or the spatulas supported by glasses to form taco shells, remove from oven and blot with the paper towel. Leave for chalupa or the tostada shells to cool flat on the pans.
5. Cool thoroughly and place for a few days in an air-tight jar. Or for up to two weeks in the refrigerator.

# Low Carb Peanut Butter Balls

**Servings:** 20

**Time:** 10 mins

**Difficulty:** Easy

**Nutrients per serving:** Calories: 104 kcal | Fat: 6g | Carbohydrates: 2g | Protein: 8g | Fiber: 1g

## Ingredients

- 1 1/3 cup whey protein powder
- 1/2 tsp stevia glycerite
- 1 cup smooth peanut butter

## Method

1. In a medium cup, add the ingredients and blend (knead) with the rubber spatula until thoroughly mixed.
2. Pinch-off sized sections of the dough with walnut and roll into the balls.
3. Up to 10 days in an airtight jar placed in the refrigerator.

# Mexican Green Beans

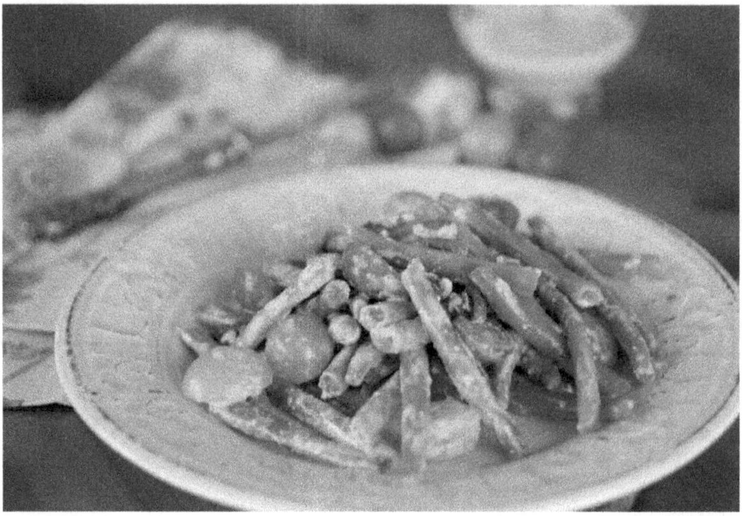

**Servings:** 6

**Time:** 25 mins

**Difficulty:** Easy

**Nutrients per serving:** Calories: 84 kcal | Fat: 7g | Carbohydrates: 6g | Protein: 1g | Fiber: 3g

## Ingredients

- 1/4 cup chopped onion (1 oz)

- 1 tsp fresh oregano, minced (or 1/4 tsp of dry but fresh tastes different)
- 1/4 tsp ground cumin
- 1/2 cup Roma tomato, seeded and diced (4 oz)
- 1 lb green beans, trimmed and cut
- 1 clove garlic, minced
- 2 tbsp avocado oil or good olive oil
- 1 tbsp butter, ghee, or another tbsp of oil
- 2 tbsp water
- 1 whole bay leaf, crumbled
- 1 tsp chicken base
- salt and pepper to taste

## Method

1. Wash the beans, strip them, and cut them. To separate seeds, split the tomato in half, squeeze carefully over the garbage, and then dice. Chop the onion, ginger, mince, and fresh oregano (if using).
2. Heat 1 tbsp of oil over medium heat in a large frying pan. Add the onion, tomato, garlic, and bay leaf when it is hot until the onion starts to soften. Add water, oil, oregano, green beans, and cumin, and for another tbsp to the chicken's base. Whisk to coat the beans and use a sheet of foil or a cap to cover them loosely. Cook for about 4 minutes or when the beans become cooked or according to your preference.
3. Apply butter, add garlic, pepper, or more oregano and the cumin to change the seasoning. Now serve.

# Broccoli Fritters With Cheddar Cheese

**Servings:** 4

**Time:** 18 mins

**Difficulty:** Easy

**Nutrients per serving:** Calories: 204 kcal | Fat: 16g | Carbohydrates: 5.8g | Protein: 12g | Fiber: 3g

## Ingredients

- 1 cup shredded cheddar cheese
- 1 Tbsp avocado oil
- 1 tsp Cajun seasoning
- 2 large eggs, beaten
- 2 Tbsp oat fiber or almond flour, or the powdered pork rinds
- 8 oz. broccoli (cut into small pieces or chopped)

## Method

1. Cut the crowns of fresh broccoli and stems into half-inch by half-inch sections. In the oven or a steamer, steam gently. If damp, remove any extra water and then dry with

paper towels. (Drain well and cut into small bite-sized bits if surplus broccoli is used.)

2. With the flour of your choosing and a Cajun seasoning, toss or swirl the broccoli to coat. Mix the egg and stir. Apply the cheddar cheese and whisk until mixed thoroughly.

3. Once heated, put a cast iron or the non-stick pan on medium heat. To oil the pan, apply the oil, and swirl. Less oil is essential for a non-stick pan. The mixture is visually separated into fourths and spooned into the tray, placed in a low mound or a patty. Back into the piles, scrape some tumbled pieces.

4. In one hand, cook until the cheese starts to melt on top of the patty and the bottom becomes crusty brown around 2-3 minutes. Flip and sear until browned on the other hand.

5. Serve with an egg or a dipping sauce on top.

# Low Carb Hamburger Buns

**Servings:** 5

**Time:** 23 mins

**Difficulty:** Easy

**Nutrients per serving:** Calories: 294 kcal | Fat: 25g | Carbohydrates: 7g | Protein: 14g | Fiber: 3g

## Ingredients

- 2 tbsp oat fiber (or protein powder or 1/4 c. more almond flour)
- 2 oz cream cheese
- 1 tbsp baking powder
- 1 large egg
- 1 1/4 cup almond flour
- 1 1/2 cup part-skim grated mozzarella cheese

## Method

1. Place the cream cheese and mozzarella cheese in a healthy microwave bowl, then microwave for about 1 minute. Whisk and microwave for an extra 30 seconds

to 1 min. Scrape the cheese along with the egg into a food processor and process until they become smooth.

2. Include the dry ingredients, then process them until they form a dough. It's pretty sticky. Let it cool for a few minutes if it's too hot to touch.
3. Preheat the oven to 400 °F. Put the rack in the center of the oven. Cover a sheet with parchment for baking. At the bottom of an oven, put a cheap metal pan.
4. Cut into 5 sections equal to each other. Lightly oil your hands and roll each piece into a ball. Place your hand on the parchment paper and softly flatten it slightly while still maintaining the domed shape.
5. At the bottom of an oven, put 6 ice cubes in a metal tray. Then the rolls are put in the oven. That will help raise and disperse the rolls.
6. Bake for about 12 minutes or until golden brown on the outside. These will be soft still, so before removing them from the baking sheet, let them cool. Store in the refrigerator after cooling. Slightly warm for pleasure.
7. Hold the burger buns in an air-tight jar in the refrigerator. They can be stored for 7-10 days and freeze well too.

# Crispy Fried Eggplant Rounds With Parmesan Cheese and Marinara Sauce

**Servings:** 4

**Time:** 30 mins

**Difficulty:** Easy

**Nutrients per serving:** Calories: 233 kcal | Fat: 17.26g | Carbohydrates: 7.15g | Protein: 11.38g | Fiber: 4g

## Ingredients

- 1 cup crushed pork rinds (1 oz/ 28.35 g)
- 1 lb eggplant (cut crosswise into 1 cm - 1/2 inch rounds, 453.6 g)
- 1 tsp dried basil
- 1 tsp dried oregano
- 1/2 cup grated Parmesan cheese (1 oz/ 28.35 g)
- 1/2 tsp salt
- 1/4 tsp granulated garlic
- 1/4 tsp onion powder
- 2 tbsp olive oil
- 2 large eggs, beaten
- 1/4 tsp pepper

## Method

1. Preparation: Put the eggplant in 10-12 rounds, sprinkle with salt, and leave to drain for 15 minutes in a colander. Dry full-on towels with paper. Meanwhile, in a shallow bowl (soup or cereal bowl), put the eggs wide enough to hold an eggplant round and scramble with the fork. In another small dish, blend the pork rinds, cheese, and seasoning. Get a little sheet pan packed.
2. Procedure: Use a fork to pick up around and flip this back and forth along the egg until fully coated. Grab a fork and let the egg fly away. Place in the crumb mixture, and crumbs cover the end. To the end, click the crumbs. Then use the fork to turn the round over and do this again. Raise the round eggplant and shake the excess crumbs. Lay yourself on a pan of paper. On all of the rounds, repeat the process. Depending on how large they are, you should've enough for 10-12 rounds.
3. Cook: Over medium-high cook, heat an iron skillet or non-stick pan. Alternatively, a large pancake skillet may be used, and both fit on the skillet at once. Add the oil when it is hot (you will need much less oil in a non-stick skillet). When the oil becomes hot, add 3-4 rounds to the pan and cook on either side for 3 minutes. To rinse, switch to a paper towel and then to a cooling rack. You may have to add a few more oil to the skillet as you go or adjust the heat just slightly. It'll be brown and crispy with the eggplant. Serve with hot mayo, tomato sauce, or serve as it is.

# Easy Low Carb Roll

**Servings:** 8

**Time:** 18 mins

**Difficulty:** Easy

**Nutrients per serving:** Calories: 165 kcal | Fat: 13g | Carbohydrates: 3g | Protein: 10g | Fiber: 1g

## Ingredients

- 2 tbsp whey protein powder (or oat fiber or coconut flour or 1/4 cup more almond flour)
- 2 oz. cream cheese, cubed
- 1 tsp baking soda (or 1 tbsp of baking powder)
- 1 large egg
- 1 1/4 cup almond flour
- 1 1/2 cup shredded skim mozzarella cheese

## Method

1. a microwave-safe dish, melt the cream cheese and mozzarella together for 1 minute at maximum strength. Stir, then heat for a further 30-45 seconds to

melt. Scrape the cheese into a food processor's bowl and process until mixed completely. Add the egg and whisk until mixed.

2. The food processor adds the dry ingredients and process until thoroughly mixed (about 10-15 seconds).
3. Using oil to spray a sheet of cling film to scrape the bread dough into the middle of the cling film. It's VERY STICKY. Shape the dough softly into a disc or oval and cool it in the freezer until the oven is ready. (NOTE: the dough doesn't have to go into the freezer if it's not sticky.)
4. Preheat an oven to 400 °F. Put the rack in the center of the oven. Line a piece of parchment or Silpat with a baking sheet.
5. Remove the dough from the freezer when the oven is ready, and cut it into 8 pieces. The dough would stick to the knife-like crazy. It's all right.
6. To flatten the rim, softly oiled your hands, carefully roll the dough portion into a ball and lower it onto the prepared cookie sheet. For the remaining dough, reverse the procedure. Sprinkle with sesame, poppy, or dehydrated onion seeds, pressing very softly to bind to the dough.
7. Bake for 13-15 minutes, roughly. It will brown the dough, and it will break. Enjoy, enjoy. Hold the extra rolls in the fridge (or freezer) and warm them gently before feeding.

# Asparagus with Hollandaise Sauce

**Servings:** 4

**Time:** 15 mins

**Difficulty:** Easy

**Nutrients per serving:** Calories: 248 kcal | Fat: 26g | Carbohydrates: 3g | Protein: 4g | Fiber: 1g

## Ingredients

- salt and pepper to taste
- 1 tbsp water
- 1 lb asparagus, trimmed

Hollandaise Sauce

- 1 tbsp water
- 1/2 tsp Dijon mustard
- 1-2 pinch cayenne pepper
- 1-2 pinch white pepper
- 1-2 tsp freshly squeezed lemon juice (or white vinegar)
- 2 large egg yolks
- 4 oz. salted butter

## Method

1. If the asparagus' thickness is medium-large, cut 1 inch from the bottom and use a vegetable peeler to gently peel the stalks. Start from the top at around 1/3 and proceed at the bottom of every spear. Keep a spear at the bottom. If the asparagus is thin, then bend it until it snaps. Split to the same length as the remaining bows. Separate the eggs for another use, reserving the whites.
2. In a microwave-safe dish, put the asparagus and add 1 tbsp of water. Cover with the plastic wrap and cook, depending on the microwave, at high power for 1 1/2 - 2 1/2 minutes. Drain the water out to leave it hidden. Alternatively, in boiling broth, blanch the asparagus until crisply tender, rinse, and keep warm.
3. In a mixer, mix the egg yolks, 1 tbsp of water, 1 tsp of lemon juice, and mustard. Put the lid on top, then remove the piece from the center. In a medium-sized to the large frying pan, put the butter and melt the butter over a medium flame. Turn the heat to medium-high and rotate the pan softly every couple of moments. Turn the heat off as the solids at the bottom of a pan start to turn brown. Turn the blender down and start pouring that hot butter in the blender, leaving behind the brown solids in the pan.
4. Add the white pepper and cayenne pepper after the butter has been absorbed, and mix. With more vinegar, salt, or pepper, change the seasoning. Pour on the asparagus and quickly eat.

# Green Beans Almondine

**Servings:** 4

**Time:** 15 mins

**Difficulty:** Easy

**Nutrients per serving:** Calories: 177 kcal | Fat: 16g | Carbohydrates: 9g | Protein: 3g | Fiber: 4g

## Ingredients

- salt and pepper to taste
- 4 tbsp butter
- 1/4 cup flaked or slivered almonds
- 1 tbsp lemon juice
- 1 lb trimmed green beans

Optional (any, not both)

- 1 clove garlic, minced
- 1 tbsp shallots, minced

## Method

1. Preparation: Wash & trim the green beans for a good appearance, cutting on the bias. Mince when using garlic or the shallots. To make squeezing simpler, roll a lemon on the table.
2. Beans: Put the green beans with 1-2 tbsp of water in the microwave-safe dish and cover with a clinging wrap. Microwave until practically crisp-tender for 2-3 minutes; the duration will depend on the microwave. Drain and stir the water. To release gas, leave it exposed.
3. Boil a pot of water and keep a big bowl of ice water standing by the Conventional method. Add the green beans while the water is boiling and cook when crisp-tender and light green. To stop frying, pour the beans and drop them directly into the ice bath. Drain them a little and dry them.
4. Over medium heat, put a large saute pan and add the almonds and butter. Cook just until the almonds have just started to brown. (Add now and mix until fragrant if using garlic cloves or shallot). Add the green beans immediately and stir in the butter to cover. All the way through, steam the beans, then squeeze lemon juice over them. To taste and serve, add salt and pepper.

# Spicy Jalapeno Coleslaw

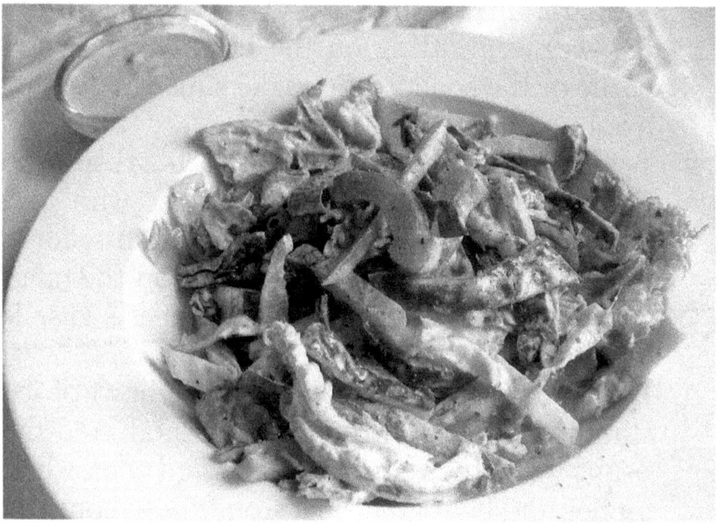

**Servings:** 10

**Time:** 15 mins

**Difficulty:** Easy

**Nutrients per serving:** Calories: 109 kcal | Fat: 10g | Carbohydrates: 4g | Protein: 1g | Fiber: 1g

## Ingredients

- ¼ cup Mayonnaise

- ¼ cup Red Bell Pepper, julienned
- ¼ cup Yellow Bell Pepper, julienned
- ½ tsp Chili powder
- 1 Jalapeno pepper, seeded and finely diced
- 1 lime, juiced
- 1 tbsp Cilantro, minced
- 1/2 cup Ranch dressing
- 2 oz. Red cabbage, finely sliced
- 8.5 oz. Coleslaw mix

**Method**

1. Toss the coleslaw mixture, red bell pepper, jalapeno pepper, and yellow bell pepper together in a big dish .

2. Mix the ranch dressing, lime juice, mayonnaise, chili powder, and cilantro in a shallow dish.

3. Using the slaw to spill the dressing over and toss to cover.

4. Until serving, refrigerate for about 30 minutes.

# Cucumber Avocado Tomato Salad

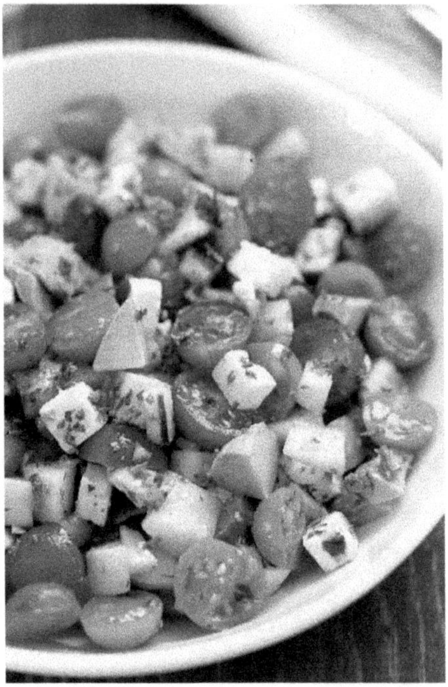

**Servings:** 10

**Time:** 15 mins

**Difficulty:** Easy

**Nutrients per serving:** Calories: 136 kcal | Fat: 12g | Carbohydrates: 8g | Protein: 2g | Fiber: 4g

## Ingredients

- ¼ cup Olive Oil
- ¼ cup Red Wine Vinegar
- ½ Red Onion
- ½ tsp Salt, plus more to taste
- 1/4 tsp Black pepper,
- 2 Avocados
- 2 large Cucumber
- 3 tbsp Lime juice
- 4 large Tomatoes

## Method

1. Cut the vegetables into bite-size pieces.
2. In a little mug, mix the olive oil, vinegar, salt, lime juice, and pepper.
3. In a wide dish, toss the cucumbers and tomatoes together and then spray the seasoning over them, turning them until all is well seasoned.
4. Add the bits of avocado and fold them carefully into the salad.
5. Immediately serve.

# Easy Pickled Cauliflower

**Servings:** 8

**Time:** 2 days 20 mins

**Difficulty:** Easy

**Nutrients per serving:** Calories: 39 kcal | Fat: 1g | Carbohydrates: 6g | Protein: 1g | Fiber: 1g

## Ingredients

- 1 small Cauliflower
- 1 cup White vinegar
- 1 cup Apple cider vinegar
- 2 cups Water
- 4 cloves Garlic
- 2 Tbsp Sugar, (or sugar substitute)
- 1 tbsp Kosher salt
- 2 tbsp Mustard seed
- 2 tsp Coriander seeds
- 1/2 Red Pepper
- 1/2 orange bell pepper
- ¼ tsp Red pepper flakes
- 2 tsp Black peppercorns

## Method

1. Divide a sliced cauliflower into 2 wide mouths pint mason jars and bell peppers equally.
2. In a small pot, add vinegar, water, garlic, sugar, coriander, mustard seeds, peppercorns, salt, and red pepper flakes and put to a boil on medium-high heat.
3. Remove it from heat until the mixture hits a boil and let it cool about 5 minutes before pouring it into each jar. Make sure that in each container, you have an equal distribution of spices.
4. Before screwing a lid on and sticking the jars in the fridge, let that mixture cool completely. Let it rest for 24 to 48 hours before eating.

# Italian Antipasto Skewers

**Servings:** 12

**Time:** 10 mins

**Difficulty:** Easy

**Nutrients per serving:** Calories: 224 kcal | Fat: 46g | Carbohydrates: 7g | Protein: 21g | Fiber: 2g

## Ingredients

- 8 oz. Primo Taglio Mozzarella Cheese
- 5 oz. Artichoke Hearts
- 3 oz.Primo Taglio Prosciutto
- 24 leaves Fresh Basil
- 2 oz. Primo Taglio Italian Sliced Salame (Dry)
- 16 oz.Roasted Red Peppers
- 12 Olives

## Method

1. Split three strips of 1/2 inch mozzarella. Cut the slices into 4 quarters each.
2. Cut 6 lengthwise artichoke hearts in half.

3. On a 5 inch skewer, arrange the ingredients. Start with a slice of salami. To form a wedge shape, fold it in half and then again in half. Push on the skewer for that.
4. thA slice of folded basil accompanies it, then a wedge of mozzarella cheese as well as the other folded basil leaf.
5. Now Cut roasted red pepper into the 1-inch wide strip 2-inch high, fold and slip onto the skewer.
6. Roll it up and cut a piece of prosciutto in two. Press it on the skewer, preceded by half of the artichoke's heart and one of the olives.

# Oven Roasted Cabbage Steaks

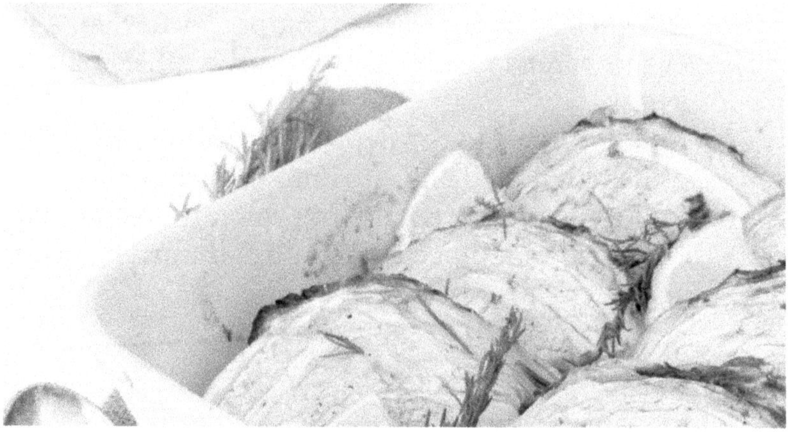

**Servings:** 6

**Time:** 40 mins

**Difficulty:** Easy

**Nutrients per serving:** Calories: 125 kcal | Fat: 10g | Carbohydrates: 9g | Protein: 3g | Fiber: 4g

## Ingredients

- 1/4 cup Olive oil
- 1 head Cabbage
- 2 tbsp Parmesan (finely grated)

- 1 clove Garlic (finely minced)
- ½ tsp Crushed red pepper flakes
- ½ tsp Kosher Salt

**Method**

1. Cut cabbage into half-inch-thick slices, then put it on a baking sheet lined with foil.
2. Mix the olive oil, parmesan cheese, garlic cracked red pepper flakes, and salt together in a shallow cup.
3. Slightly covering each side, brush the mixture on the cabbage slices.
4. Bake for 15 minutes in an oven at 400°F. Flip the slices of cabbage and finish baking for a full 15 minutes.

# Keto Colcannon

**Servings:** 12

**Time:** 15 mins

**Difficulty:** Easy

**Nutrients per serving:** Calories: 58 kcal | Fat: 4g | Carbohydrates: 5g | Protein: 2g | Fiber: 2g

## Ingredients

- Salt to taste
- 6 oz. cabbage (cut into thin 1-inch long slices)
- 4 tbsp butter, divided
- 36 oz. Cauliflower, chopped

## Method

1. To a simmer, put a big pot of water. Add the cauliflower and let it simmer for 10 minutes or so. You will feel that when it is soft to quickly split off with a fork, the cauliflower is finished.

2. Melt 1 tbsp of butter in the large skillet while the cauliflower is cooking. Include the cabbage and saute until softened for 5-7 minutes.

3. When the cauliflower has done frying, pour the water into a strainer and rinse it thoroughly. To eliminate water as possible, let it stay for several minutes .

4. In the empty cup, pour a cauliflower back in and add cabbage and the leftover butter. Marinate together until the consistency of mashed potato.

5. To taste, apply salt and serve.

# Keto Blueberry Scones

**Servings:** 8

**Time:** 33 mins

**Difficulty:** Easy

**Nutrients per serving:** Calories: 110 kcal | Fat: 8g | Carbohydrates: 6g | Protein: 2g | Fiber: 2g

## Ingredients

- 3/4 cup Almond flour
- 1/4 cup Coconut flour
- 1/4 tsp salt
- 1/4 cup butter, unsalted, softened
- 1/4 cup Almond Milk (Unsweetened)
- 5 tbsp Granular erythritol sweetener
- 2 tsp gluten-free baking powder
- 2 tsp Vanilla extract
- 1 large Egg
- 1 cup Blueberries

## Method

1. Preheat the oven to 350 °F.
2. Mix all the dry ingredients in the bowl of your blender (except the chocolate chips).
3. Include the softened butter and milk it until it is well combined and there are no bits of butter along with the dry ingredients.
4. Include the vanilla extract, almond milk, and egg and begin combining until well mixed.
5. Apply the blueberries and then roll them into the dough using a spatula.
6. Shape 2.5 oz of dough into a triangle shape with your palm. Place a cookie sheet on an unoiled one. Repeat until you consume all of the dough. Approximately 8 scones you can receive.
7. Bake for 18-23 minutes or when the sides are golden brown in the oven at 350 °F. You start to see some golden brown patches on top.
8. Takeout from the oven and leave to fully cool the scones before placing them in an airtight jar.

# Cheesy Bacon Brussels Sprouts

**Servings:** 6

**Time:** 35 mins

**Difficulty:** Easy

**Nutrients per serving:** Calories: 261 kcal | Fat: 23g | Carbohydrates: 8g | Protein: 8g | Fiber: 3g

## Ingredients

- 6 slices cooked bacon, chopped
- 4 tbsp Olive oil
- 2 oz. Cheddar cheese
- 1.25 tsp salt, divided
- 1 lb Brussels sprouts
- ½ tsp Onion powder
- ½ tsp Garlic powder
- ½ cup Heavy cream
- ¼ tsp Salt

## Method

1. Preheat the oven to 375° F.

2. Over medium heat, heat a large size oven-safe skillet.
3. Add the olive oil and the sprouts from Brussels. Sprinkle with 1 tsp of salt and simmer until the sprouts appear to soften and brown in patches, for about 10 minutes.
4. Mix the heavy cream, garlic powder, onion powder, and the remaining 1/4 tsp of salt as the brussels sprouts become cooked.
5. Remove them from the sun until the Brussels sprouts are prepared and pour a heavy cream mixture on them.
6. Sprinkle the Brussels sprouts with cheddar cheese and bacon over them.
7. Place the skillet in an oven until the cheese is fully melted and bake for 10 minutes.

# Keto Chocolate Chip Scones

**Servings:** 8

**Time:** 30 mins

**Difficulty:** Easy

**Nutrients per serving:** Calories: 156 kcal | Fat: 20g | Carbohydrates: 5g | Protein: 2g | Fiber: 2g

## Ingredients

- 4.5 oz. Lily's Dark Chocolate Chips
- 3/4 cup Almond flour
- 1/4 cup Coconut flour
- 1/4 tsp salt
- 1/4 cup butter, unsalted, softened
- 1/4 cup Unsweetened Almond Milk
- 5 tbsp Granular erythritol sweetener
- 2 tsp gluten-free baking powder
- 2 tsp Vanilla extract
- 1 large Egg

## Method

1. Preheat the oven to 350 °F.
2. Mix all of the dry ingredients in the bowl of your blender (except for the chocolate chips).
3. Apply the softened butter and milk it until it is well combined, and there are no bits of butter along with the dry ingredients.
4. Apply the vanilla extract, almond milk, and egg and begin combining until well mixed.
5. Include the chocolate chips and then roll them into the dough using a spatula.
6. Shape 2.5 oz of dough into a triangle shape with your palm. Place a cookie sheet on an unoiled one. Repeat until you consume all of the dough. Approximately 8 scones you can receive.
7. Bake for 17-21 minutes or until the sides are golden brown in the 350 °F ovens, and you have to see golden brown patches on top. Remove from the oven and leave to fully cool the scones before placing them in an airtight jar.

# Classic Cheese Ball Recipe

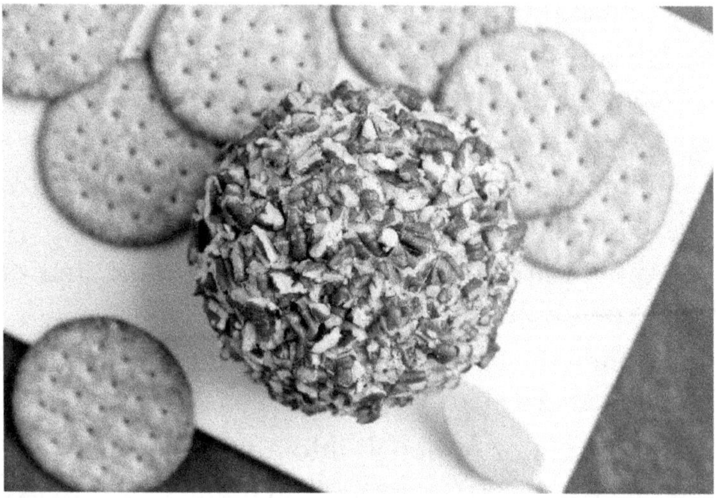

**Servings:** 10

**Time:** 10 mins

**Difficulty:** Easy

**Nutrients per serving:** Calories: 238 kcal | Fat: 22g | Carbohydrates: 3g | Protein: 8g | Fiber: 1g

## Ingredients

- 8 oz. Cream Cheese, softened
- 8 oz. Cheddar Cheese shredded

- 2 tsp Worcestershire sauce
- 1 tsp Lemon juice
- 1 tsp Green onion, finely chopped
- 1 cup Pecans, roughly chopped
- ¼ tsp Salt

**Method**

1. 1.In the bowl of the stand mixer, put the cream cheese, green onion, cheddar cheese, Worcestershire sauce, salt, lemon juice, and blend until all the ingredients are thoroughly mixed.
2. Scrape the bowl with the mixture and shape it into a ball.
3. Use the chopped pecans to roll the ball until it is completely enclosed.
4. Cover the ball of cheese in plastic wrap and put for 1 hour in the refrigerator to cool.
5. Serve with crackers and vegetables.

# Air Fryer Chicken Wings

**Servings:** 4

**Time:** 40 mins

**Difficulty:** Easy

**Nutrients per serving:** Calories: 375 kcal | Fat: 31g | Carbohydrates: 1g | Protein: 23g | Fiber: 1g

## Ingredients

- 1 tsp Pepper
- 1/2 cup Frank's Red Hot Sauce
- 1/4 cup butter, melted
- 2 lb Chicken wings (cut into drumettes and flat)
- 2 tsp salt

## Method

1. Pat's chicken drumettes and the wings dry with a paper towel and put them on the baking sheet or a cutting board.
2. Sprinkle salt and pepper on the chicken.

3. Put the chicken in an air-fryer basket and cook for 25 minutes at 380 °F. Cut the basket halfway through and use tongs to dip the chicken around and shift it around so that bottom reaches the top.
4. Turn the heat to 400 °F after 25 minutes and continue cooking for 5 minutes or when the skin is crispy.
5. Take the chicken from the basket and put it in a wide bowl with the fryer.
6. Over the chicken wings, add the sauce and throw them until well seasoned.
7. Immediately serve.

# Instant Pot Turnip Greens & Collard Greens

**Servings:** 6

**Time:** 20 mins

**Difficulty:** Easy

**Nutrients per serving:** Calories: 256 kcal | Fat: 23g | Carbohydrates: 8g | Protein: 3g | Fiber: 3g

## Ingredients

- 20 oz. Turnip greens or collard greens (stem removed and roughly chopped)
- 1 cup Chicken broth
- ½ cup Onion, diced
- 2 tbsp Vinegar
- Salt and pepper to taste
- 6 oz. Salt pork (diced into about 1/4-inch pieces)

**Method**

1. Set the Instant pot to saute, add pork or bacon salt and onions, and cook until the pork is crisp and the onions become softened.
2. Pour the chicken broth into a pot and deglaze the pan's bottle to ensure the browned bits get up. To stop the saute feature, click cancel.
3. In the greens, add some vinegar and the package so that the pot is around 2/3 of the way finished.
4. Lock the lid and turn the valve to the SEALING position. For 10 minutes, set to high Intensity.
5. When the timer goes off, adjust the valve to Ventilation and let all the air out by rapidly opening it.
6. To blend it, remove the lid, swirl the pot's contents, and apply salt and black pepper.

# Keto Avocado Coleslaw

**Servings:** 8

**Time:** 10 mins

**Difficulty:** Easy

**Nutrients per serving:** Calories: 123 kcal | Fat: 10g | Carbohydrates: 8g | Protein: 2g | Fiber: 4g

## Ingredients

- 1/2 cup Sour Cream
- 1/2 tsp salt
- 16 oz. Coleslaw mix (or shredded cabbage)
- 2 Avocado
- 3-4 tbsp Lime Juice (more to taste)

## Method

1. Stir mixture into coleslaw.
2. Mash avocado with sour cream, lime juice, and salt.
3. Keep refrigerated until you are ready to serve.

# Buffalo Chicken Jalapeño Poppers

**Servings:** 8

**Time:** 50 mins

**Difficulty:** Easy

**Nutrients per serving:** Calories: 408 kcal | Fat: 33g | Carbohydrates: 4g | Protein: 21g

## Ingredients

Buffalo Chicken Dip

- 8 oz. Cream Cheese, softened
- 3 tbsp Ranch Dressing
- 2 Chicken Breasts (approximately 12 oz.)
- 1/2 cup Frank's Red Hot sauce
- 1/2 cup Cheddar Cheese, (shredded)

Buffalo Chicken Jalapeño Poppers (Make Almost 30 Poppers)

- 16-20 Jalapeños, halved
- 16-20 Strips Bacon
- Buffalo Chicken Dip,

**Method**

Buffalo Chicken Dip

1. Boil the water.
2. For 15 minutes, or when cooked through, put the chicken breasts in the boiling water.
3. Remove the chicken breasts and insert them directly in the mixing bowl of the stand mixer. (You should use the fork to shred a chicken by hand if you do not have a stand mixer.)
4. Turn the mixer to medium for about 1-2 minutes or until the chicken is entirely shredded using a dough hook. To make sure all the chicken becomes shredded, stir once or twice.
5. Transfer the chicken to the softened cream cheese and mix it thoroughly.
6. Apply the hot sauce and thoroughly mix.
7. Include the ranch and shredded cheese and mix thoroughly.

Buffalo Chicken Jalapeño Poppers

1. Preheat the oven to 400° F.
2. Cook bacon partly, making it partly crisp but still flexible enough to coil around the poppers.
3. With a heaping tbsp of buffalo chicken sauce, stuff the jalapeno halves with it.
4. Wrap a slice of bacon for each jalapeño popper.
5. On a baking sheet, place the stuffed poppers.
6. Bake until the jalapeños are softened, and the bacon is crispy in the oven. 20 minutes roughly.

# Low Carb Big Mac Bites

**Servings:** 16

**Time:** 35 mins

**Difficulty:** Easy

**Nutrients per serving:** Calories: 182 kcal | Fat: 12g | Carbohydrates: 1g | Protein: 10g

## Ingredients

- ¼ cup Onion, finely diced
- 1 tsp salt
- 1.5 lb Ground beef
- 16 slices Dill Pickle
- 4 slices American Cheese
- Lettuce

<u>SECRET SAUCE</u>

- 1 tsp Garlic powder
- 1 tsp Onion powder
- 1 tsp Paprika
- 1 tsp White wine vinegar
- 1/2 cup Mayonnaise
- 2 tbsp yellow mustard

- 4 tbsp Dill pickle relish

## Method

1. Preheat the oven to 400°F.
2. Mix the onions, ground beef, and salt in a large dish. Mix when mixed thoroughly.
3. Roll the beef into balls of 1.5 oz.. To make the mini burger patty, press every one slightly down to flatten it and put it on the lined baking sheet.
4. Now Bake for 15 minutes or until fully baked at 400 °F.
5. When cooking burgers, add all the secret sauce components to a bowl and mix to blend.
6. Switch off the oven when the burgers baking finished and remove them—Pat off the extra oil.
7. Cut four squares of each cheese slice and put a square on each mini-patty. Place the cheese back in the oven and let it melt.
8. Place a few lettuces (squares) and a pickle slice on top of each meatball, and drive a skewer through it. Serve or have the special sauce.

# Ranch Baked Pork Chops

**Servings:** 4

**Time:** 35 mins

**Difficulty:** Easy

**Nutrients per serving:** Calories: 252 kcal | Fat: 9g | Carbohydrates: 7g | Protein: 32g

## Ingredients

- 4 Pork Chops, 1 inch thick
- 2 tsp Dried Parsley
- 2 tsp Garlic Powder
- 2 tsp Paprika
- 1 tsp Dried Dill Weed
- 1 tsp Dried Minced Onions
- 1 tsp Sea Salt
- ½ tsp Dried Chives
- ½ tsp Onion Powder
- 1/2 tsp Ground Black Pepper
- 1/4 cup Dry Buttermilk Powder

## Method

1. Preheat the oven to 400°F.
2. To make the ranch seasoning, add all the dry ingredients in the bowl and blend thoroughly.
3. In the ranch seasoning, dip each pork chop, turning it over when it is thoroughly coated. Before lying on a baking sheet, shake off the residue.
4. In the oven, put the pork chops and bake for 15 to 25 minutes. When it touches an internal temperature of 145 °F, the pork chop is cooked.
5. Until eating, let the pork chops rest for about 5 minutes.

# Low Carb Nachos

**Servings:** 8

**Time:** 35 mins

**Difficulty:** Easy

**Nutrients per serving:** Calories: 227 kcal | Fat: 14g | Carbohydrates: 6g | Protein: 18g | Fiber: 1g

## Ingredients

- Toppings such as avocado, sour cream, tomatoes,
- 8 oz Cheddar Cheese (shredded)
- 20 Mini Sweet Peppers (halved and seeded)
- 2 tbsp Chili Powder
- 1/2 tsp salt
- 1 tbsp Cumin
- 1 lb Ground Beef, chicken, steak, or pork, cooked
- 1 Jalapeno, sliced

**Method**

1. Cook your favorite meat in a skillet, adding cumin, chili powder, and salt. On a sheet plate, put the mini sweet pepper halves.
2. Sprinkle the cooked meat over the mini peppers and hold it in peppers to spill into the pan. Cover the mini peppers with jalapeno slices and shredded cheese.
3. Put in a BROIL-set oven for about 5-6 minutes or when the cheese is completely melted.
4. Apply some low carb toppings you need for the nacho.

# Air Fryer Low Carb Mozzarella Sticks

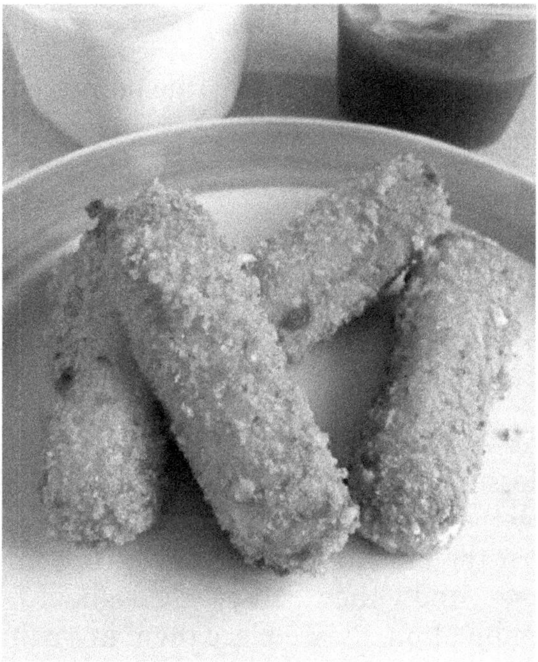

**Servings:** 6

**Time:** 20 mins

**Difficulty:** Easy

**Nutrients per serving:** Calories: 267 kcal | Fat: 20g | Carbohydrates: 4g | Protein: 18g | Fiber: 1g

## Ingredients

- 1 tsp Italian seasoning
- 1/2 cup Almond flour
- 1/2 cup Parmesan cheese (the powdered form)
- 1/2 tsp Garlic Salt
- 12 Mozzarella sticks, string cheese (cut in half)
- 2 large eggs, beaten

## Method

1. Mix the almond flour, Italian seasoning, parmesan cheese, and garlic salt in a dish. Whisk the eggs together in a separate dish.
2. Coat the mozzarella stick halves in your egg one at a time and then toss throughout the coating combination. Please place them in a suitable jar.
3. Place parchment paper among the mozzarella sticks layers if you need to make more than 1 sheet. Freeze for 30 minutes the sticks of mozzarella
4. Remove it from the freezer and placed it in the Philips AirFryer.
5. Adjust to 400 °F for 5 minutes and cook.
6. Open the air fryer and then let for 1 min before moving to a plate of low carbohydrate mozzarella sticks.

# Crab Cakes With Roasted Red Pepper Sauce

**Servings:** 8

**Time:** 40 mins

**Difficulty:** Easy

**Nutrients per serving:** Calories: 65 kcal | Fat: 4g | Carbohydrates: 4g | Protein: 6g

## Ingredients

- 2 tsp Old Bay seasoning
- 2 tsp dijon mustard
- 2 Tbsp parsley, chopped
- 2 Tbsp coconut oil
- 1.5 Tbsp coconut flour
- 1 Tbsp fresh lemon juice
- 1 egg, beaten
- 1 cup lump crab meat

**Method**

1. 1.Pick the crab carefully to ensure the absence of shells or the cartilage in meat and add it to a small bowl. Mix the lemon juice, egg, and dijon mustard in another small cup, blending until smooth.
2. Mix the parsley, old bay, and coconut flour in a third dish, stirring thoroughly. Add the mixture of eggs to the crab softly, folding when mixed. Then apply to the crab mixture the dry ingredients and gently blend in. Try not to cut up the crab bits or shred them too far.
3. Heat the coconut oil in a nonstick saute pan over medium heat. Create 8 small cakes and carefully put them in the hot oil. Cook on either side for around 2-3 minutes, or until golden brown. Move to a plate lined with paper towels from the dish.
4. Sprinkle with kosher salt and serve with the Roasted Red Pepper Sauce and half squeeze a fresh lemon over it.

# Low Carb Taco Bites

**Servings:** 30

**Time:** 1 hr

**Difficulty:** Easy

**Nutrients per serving:** Calories: 73 kcal | Fat: 5g | Carbohydrates: 1g | Protein: 4g

## Ingredients

- Pico de Gallo for garnish
- 8 tsp Sour Cream for garnish
- 2 tbsp Cumin
- 2 tbsp Chili Powder
- 2 cup Packaged Shredded Cheddar Cheese
- 1 tsp salt + more to taste
- 1 lb Ground Beef

## Method

1. Preheat the oven to 350 °F. Place 1 tbsp pile of cheese 2 inches apart on the baking sheet lined with a silicone or mat parchment paper

2. Place the baking sheet in an oven and bake until the edges of cheese become brown, or for 5-7 minutes.
3. Let that cheese cool for 1 min, then pick it up and press it down into a mini muffin tin cup to shape a cup.
4. Let the cheese fully cool, and then cut it.
5. As you begin to bake the cheese and make your cups, over medium-high heat heating, put the ground beef in the skillet until it is fully cooked.
6. Drain the beef from the fat and then add 1/4 c of water and the spices.
7. Stir once mixed, then add some more salt to taste and boil for 5 minutes.
8. For cheese cups, substitute meat and finish each with 1/4 tsp of sour cream. If you like, you can also include fresh pico de gallo as well.

# Bacon Cheese Balls

**Servings:** 24

**Time:** 10 mins

**Difficulty:** Easy

**Nutrients per serving:** Calories: 89 kcal | Fat: 8g | Carbohydrates: 1g | Protein: 2g

## Ingredients

- 10 slices bacon (finely chopped)
- 4 oz. Cheddar cheese (shredded)
- 4 oz. Salted Almonds (chopped)
- 8 oz. Cream cheese

## Method

1. In a dish, mix the first 3 ingredients.
2. Roll the cheese mixture in 1-inch balls and roll and widen the ends slightly to gently mold them in an oval shape.

# Shrimp Cocktail Deviled Eggs

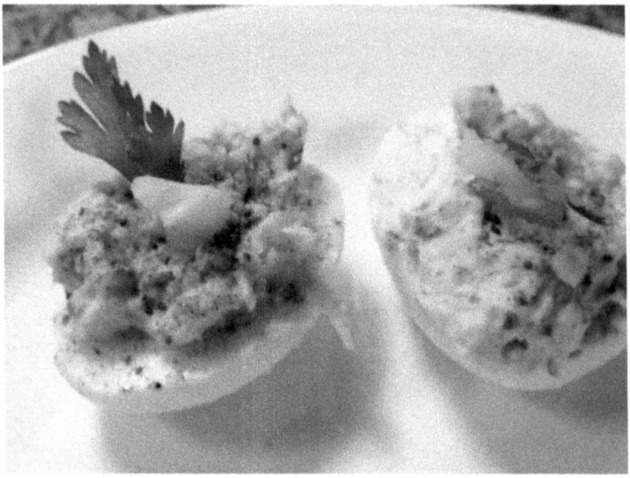

**Servings:** 12

**Time:** 30 mins

**Difficulty:** Easy

**Nutrients per serving:** Calories: 142 kcal | Fat: 11g | Carbohydrates: 1g | Protein: 8g

## Ingredients

- 1 1/2 tsp Horseradish
- 1/2 cup Mayonnaise

- 12 eggs, hard-boiled & peeled
- 24 Shrimp, steamed
- 3 tbsp Ketchup
- Paprika for garnish
- Salt to taste

## Method

1. Put the eggs in half and place the yolks in a different bowl to remove them.
2. Apply the yolks to the horseradish, mayonnaise, ketchup, and salt and mix until creamy.
3. In a piping bag, put the yolk mixture and pipe in the egg halves.
4. Place a shrimp over each shell. Garnish with Paprika.

# Shrimp Pil Pil

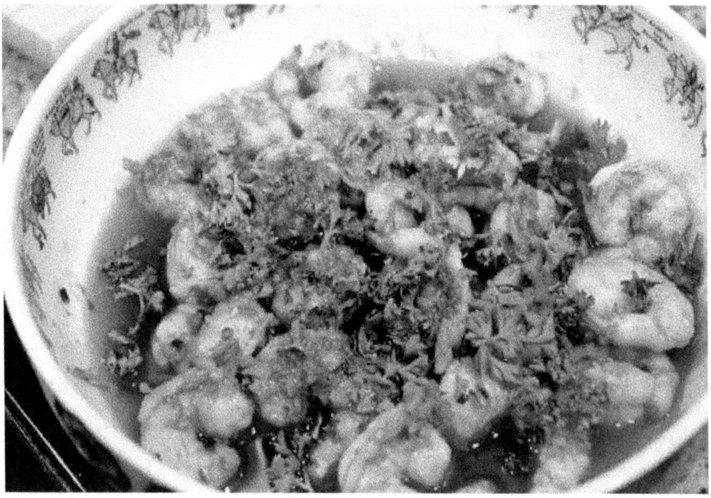

**Servings:** 8

**Time:** 10 mins

**Difficulty:** Easy

**Nutrients per serving:** Calories: 275 kcal | Fat: 25g | Carbohydrates: 2g | Protein: 14g | Fiber: 2g

## Ingredients

- 1 lb Shrimp, large (around 30 shrimp)
- 5 tbsp Butter

- 4 tbsp Tabasco
- 1 tbsp Spanish paprika
- 1 tsp Salt
- 2/3 c Olive oil

**Method**

1. Mix in the olive oil, sugar, Tabasco, paprika, and salt.
2. Place each ramekin with 3-4 shrimp and many slices of garlic.
3. Until the shrimp is partially covered, add the sauce in.
4. Put the ramekins on the baking sheet and broil them for 4-5 minutes in the oven or until the shrimp's oil bubbles and the shrimp become pink.
5. Remove from the oven and serve when hot.

# Easy Guacamole

**Servings:** 12

**Time:** 40 mins

**Difficulty:** Easy

**Nutrients per serving:** Calories: 178 kcal | Fat: 15g | Carbohydrates: 14g | Protein: 3g | Fiber: 8g

## Ingredients

- 1 Roma or vine tomato
- 1/4 cup chopped fresh cilantro
- 1/4 cup chopped red onion
- 1-2 jalapeño or serrano chilis
- 2 ripe avocados
- 2-3 limes
- sea salt

## Method

1. Peel and pit the avocado and cut the onion thinly, and add it to a dish. Mush up the entire avocado with a fork.

2. Drop the seeds and the liquid, wash and slice the tomato into half, then dice just the flesh and return it to the cup.
3. Wash and spin fresh cilantro dry and cut when you have around 1/4 cup of cilantro chopped and return it to the dish.
4. Season with lime juice and sea salt, stir it together well, and serve
5. Add freshly chopped chili to the hot guacamole, too.

# Keto Parmesan Roasted Broccoli

**Servings:** 5

**Time:** 30 mins

**Difficulty:** Easy

**Nutrients per serving:** Calories: 157 kcal | Fat: 13.8g | Carbohydrates: 4.5g | Protein: 5.5g | Fiber: 2.2g

## Ingredients

- 3 Tbsp. salted butter, melted
- 2 Tbsp. avocado oil
- 1/3 cup grated Parmesan cheese
- 1/2 tsp. salt
- 1/2 tsp. garlic powder
- 1 lb fresh broccoli florets
- 1 1/2 tsp. lemon pepper

## Method

1. Line and set aside a sheet pan with the parchment. Preheat the oven to 400°F.

2. Place the florets of the broccoli in a wide dish. Mix the melted butter, avocado oil, garlic powder, lemon pepper, and salt in a separate bowl and mix.
3. Drizzle over the broccoli with the butter mixture and toss to mix. Sprinkle the broccoli with parmesan and flip to cover it.
4. On the ready sheet pan, put the broccoli into a single layer. Bake for about 20-25 minutes or until it is soft and golden brown.

# Spicy Sautéed Mushrooms with Anchovy

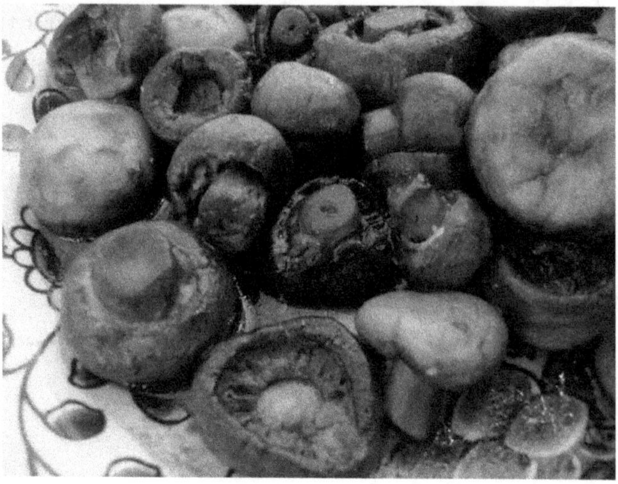

**Servings:** 4

**Time:** 20 mins

**Difficulty:** Easy

**Nutrients per serving:** Calories: 111 kcal | Fat: 8g | Carbohydrates: 9g | Protein: 3g | Fiber: 3g

## Ingredients

- Juice from 1 lemon optional
- 3 garlic cloves minced

- 2 tbsp butter or ghee
- 2 medium anchovy fillets
- 1 lb mixed mushrooms
- ¼ tsp red pepper flakes

## Method

1. Heat butter over medium-high heat in a large skillet. Apply the pepper flakes, anchovies, and garlic, as the butter melts and the foam subsides and cooked, splitting the anchovy fillets with a wooden spoon before the mixture is fragrant (approx 1 minute).
2. Include the mushrooms and cook for about 12 minutes, stirring regularly, until the mushrooms' liquid disappears and the mushrooms are finely browned. Season to taste with salt, squeeze one lemon juice (if used), and serve immediately.

# Keto Cheese Crackers

**Servings:** 11

**Time:** 30 mins

**Difficulty:** Easy

**Nutrients per serving:** Calories: 183 kcal | Fat: 17g | Carbohydrates: 4g | Protein: 6g | Fiber: 2g

## Ingredients

- 5 Tbsp. butter salted & softened
- 4 oz. Pepper Jack cheese shredded
- 2 Tbsp. coconut flour
- 1 oz cream cheese softened
- 1 cup almond flour
- ¼ tsp. Salt
- ¼ tsp. Onion powder
- ¼ tsp. Garlic powder
- ¼ tsp. cumin
- ¼ cup finely chopped pecans

## Method

1. Cream together the butter and cream cheese in the tank of the stand mixer. Apply the melted cheese and blend until mixed properly. Add the 6 ingredients, then continue blending. Stir the chopped pecans together.
2. Layer dough in plastic wrap and shape around 2 1/2 inches thick into a roll. Tightly cover-up and cool or freeze until solid.
3. Cut the chilled dough into 1/4' thick slices and put on a sheet pan lined with parchment. Bake for 20-25 minutes at 300 °F or until softly golden brown. Before withdrawing, cool crackers entirely in pots.

# Cheesy Squash Bites

**Servings:** 28

**Time:** 30 mins

**Difficulty:** Easy

**Nutrients per serving:** Calories: 76 kcal | Fat: 6g | Carbohydrates: 2g | Protein: 3g | Fiber: 1g

## Ingredients

- 4 Tbsp. butter melted
- 3 Tbsp. coconut flour
- 3 eggs
- 2 Tbsp. sour cream
- 2 cloves garlic finely minced
- 2 ½ tsp. baking powder
- 1/2 tsp. Monkfruit or Erythritol Blend Sweetener
- 1 tsp. salt
- 1 Tbsp. chopped parsley
- 1 Tbsp. butter
- 1 cup almond flour
- 1 ½ cup shredded squash
- ½ tsp. Pepper
- ½ cup Colby or Medium Cheddar cheese

- ¼ tsp. Fiesta Brand-Zesty Italian Delight/Italian Seasoning
- ¼ cup shredded Parmesan
- ¼ cup diced onion

## Method

1. Spray and set aside a mini muffin tin or fill a mini muffin tin with liners. Spray well and put aside if you are using the silicone mini muffin tray.
2. Melt one tbsp of butter in a shallow pan. Garnish with cabbage, rubbed squash, ginger, and 1/2 tsp. Add salt and sauté for 5-7 minutes, just until the onion is shiny. Put aside to cool. There should not be any liquid in the container.
3. Mix the flour and the next 6 ingredients in a large bowl and mix well to combine. Mix the eggs one at a time. Apply a mixture of melted butter, squash, and sour cream and mix well. Stir the cheese in.
4. Drop the entire tbsp or put the dough in a ready mini muffin pan using a cookie scoop.
5. For 20 minutes, bake at 350 F or until the tops are only golden brown. Cool for 5 minutes in a pan, then remove from the pan and cool thoroughly on a rack. They can be eaten warm and also store at room temperature.

# Roasted Cauliflower Keto Hummus with Red Peppers

**Servings:** 10

**Time:** 45 mins

**Difficulty:** Easy

**Nutrients per serving:** Calories: 137 kcal | Fat: 12g | Carbohydrates: 5g | Protein: 3g | Fiber: 2g

**Ingredients**

For the Roasted Cauliflower

- 3-4 Tbsp. olive (or avocado oil)
- 1 large head cauliflower (cut into florets)
- ½ tsp. Garlic powder
- ½ tsp. cumin
- 1 tsp. salt

To Finish the Hummus:

- 2-5 Tbsp. water
- 2 Tbsp. olive or avocado oil
- 2 Tbsp. fresh lemon juice
- 1-2 cloves garlic

- 1/2 tsp. Cumin
- ¾ tsp. Salt
- ¼ tsp. Pepper
- ¼ cup roasted red pepper
- ¼ cup + 2 Tbsp. tahini

## Method

1. Preheat the oven to 400°C. Toss the cauliflower florets with olive oil, garlic powder, salt, and cumin in a large cup. Load it onto a sheet pan lined with parchment. Be sure to hit the pan with all the florets for full caramelization. For 30-35 minutes, roast the cauliflower or until the florets become brown and very tender. 5-10 minutes to cool.
2. Mix the roasted cauliflower, tahini, lemon juice, and the next 6 ingredients in a food processor or the high-speed blender. Puré the mixture until it is smooth. Add a tbsp of water at a time if the hummus is too dense to achieve the target consistency. Serve with keto crackers or vegetables.

# Keto Spinach Balls

**Servings:** 16

**Time:** 30 mins

**Difficulty:** Easy

**Nutrients per serving:** Calories: 96 kcal | Fat: 8g | Carbohydrates: 1g | Protein: 5g | Fiber: 1g

## Ingredients

- 1/3 cup red onion finely minced
- 1/3 cup parmesan cheese (finely shredded)
- 1 Tbsp. butter
- 3 cloves garlic (finely minced)
- 1 cup pork rind crumbs
- 1 tsp. kosher salt
- ¼ tsp. poultry seasoning
- 10 oz. frozen spinach (squeezed dried & thawed)
- ½ cup fontina cheese (finely shredded)
- ¼ tsp. Black pepper
- 1 Tbsp. heavy cream
- 5 Tbsp. butter salted melted
- 3 eggs

**Method**

1. Preheat the oven to 350°F. Line up and set aside a large sheet pan.
2. Melt the butter in a small skillet on medium heat. Include the onion then sauté until soft and translucent for 5-7 minutes or when solid. Add garlic and simmer for an additional minute. Remove from the sun and place to cool aside.
3. Mix the dried spinach, cooled onion, pork rind crumbs, garlic, and the next eight ingredients in a medium mixing dish. Mix well and let the mixture sit for 5-10 minutes in the fridge.
4. Divide the mixture into 16 portions using a small scoop, and use your hands to shape each part into a ball. Place balls about an inch apart on the lined cookie sheet and bake for about 15-20 minutes or until they are golden. Take from a sheet pan and put to cool on paper towels. Serve at room temperature or hotter.

# Cajun Pork Rinds

**Servings:** 14

**Time:** 1 hr 13 mins

**Difficulty:** Easy

**Nutrients per serving:** Calories: 51 kcal | Fat: 5g | Carbohydrates: 1g | Protein: 1g | Fiber: 1g

## Ingredients

- 6 Tbsp. melted butter
- 2 Tbsp. Worcestershire Sauce gluten-free
- 2 3.25 oz bags of plain pork rinds
- 1/8 tsp. cayenne pepper
- 1/2 tsp. paprika
- 1/2 tsp. onion powder
- 1/2 tsp. garlic powder
- 1 1/4 tsp. Fiesta Brand-Cajun All Seasoning

## Method

1. Preheat to 250 F in the oven. Line up and set aside a large sheet pan lined with parchment.

2. Through a large dish, pour the pork rinds. In a small cup, mix the next 7 ingredients and blend well to mix. Drizzle over the pork rinds with half the butter mixture and toss to cover. Repeat with the mixture of butter that remains. Cover the coasted pork rinds over the pan of prepared sheets and bake for 80 minutes at 250 F, stirring after every 20 minutes.
3. Take the pork rinds from the oven and pass them to paper towels to make cool. When cold, place at room temperature in an air-tight bag.

# Jalapeno Stuffed Hamburger Steak Bites

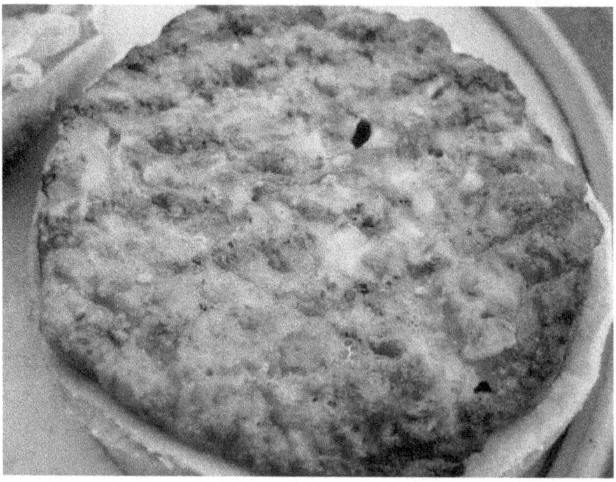

**Servings:** 8

**Time:** 25 mins

**Difficulty:** Easy

**Nutrients per serving:** Calories: 262 kcal | Fat: 23g | Carbohydrates: 2g | Protein: 10g | Fiber: 1g

## Ingredients

For an Avocado Ranch:

- 2 tsp. of Worcestershire sauce

- 1/3 cup of avocado
- 1 tsp. of creole mustard
- 1 clove garlic
- 1 ½ tsp. Hot sauce
- ½ tsp. salt
- ½ Tbsp. parsley (Dried)
- ½ cup unsweetened almond milk
- ½ cup mayonnaise
- ¼ tsp. Onion powder
- ½ tsp. of Italian seasoning

For Steak Bites:

- 2 tsp. Worcestershire Sauce
- 1 tsp. salt
- 1 lb ground beef 80/20
- 1 fresh jalapeno (seeded, deveined and finely diced)
- ½ tsp. Garlic powder
- ½ tsp. Fiesta Brand Fajita Seasoning (Salt-Free)
- ¼ tsp. black pepper
- ¼ cup purple onion (finely diced)

## Method

Avocado Ranch preparation:

1. In the blender, first mix the mayo and then the next 8 ingredients and mix until smooth and blended. Whisk in the dried herbs and pour into a cup, cover, and cool before ready to eat.

Steak Bites preparation:

1. Cut off the ground beef in the medium mixing bowl, and then add the next seven ingredients. Mix softly, blending all the meat with the seasoning and vegetables. The meat mixture or even the steak bites would be dense. You wouldn't want to over mix or execute more. Divide the mixture into 8 pieces equally, roll each potion softly into a ball, and then flatten it to around 1⁄4 inch thick. For all 8 parts, repeat.
2. Over medium-high heat, preheat the heavy skillet. Add up the 4 patties and cook for around 3 minutes/side or achieve the ideal point.
3. Serve hot with the Ranch Avocado

# Roasted Cauliflower with Chili Lime & Browned Better

**Servings:** 4

**Time:** 40 mins

**Difficulty:** Easy

**Nutrients per serving:** Calories: 207 kcal | Fat: 18g | Carbohydrates: 9g | Protein: 3g | Fiber: 3g

## Ingredients

- 6 Tbsp. butter melted
- 1/2 Tbsp. kosher salt
- 1/2 fresh lime
- 1 tsp. chili powder
- 1 head fresh cauliflower, dried
- 1 dash -1/8 tsp cayenne pepper
- ½ Tbsp. Granulated garlic
- ¼ tsp. cumin
- ¼ tsp paprika

**Method**

1. Preheat the oven to 425 °F and set aside a sheet pan with the lined-parchment.
2. Place the florets of the cauliflower in a wide cup. In a small bowl and wick, mix melted butter and the other 6 ingredients to combine. Toss the butter and spices with the florets until they are fully covered.
3. Disperse the florets on the ready sheet pan and bake for 25 to 30 minutes at 425 °F or until the florets become golden brown; whisk during the baking period. Remove from the oven and strain the florets with fresh lime. Now immediately serve.

- Freshly ground black pepper
- Diamond Crystal kosher salt
- avocado oil (or cooking fat of choice)
- 5 medium portobello mushrooms
- 2 tbsp ghee (or fat of choice)
- 1½ cups marinara sauce
- 1 tbsp coconut flour
- 1 lb uncooked sausage (removed from its casing)
- 1 large egg lightly beaten
- ½ small onion minced
- ½ lb frozen spinach (defrosted & squeezed dried)

Lightning Source UK Ltd.
Milton Keynes UK
UKHW020214080521
383350UK00003B/292